The Complete Calorie Counter

Also in Pan Books

The Complete Carbohydrate Counter
with an introduction by Katie Stewart

compiled by Kyle Cathie
with an introduction by
Eileen Fowler MBE

The complete
calorie counter

Pan Original Pan Books

First published 1976 by Pan Books Ltd,
Cavaye Place, London SW10 9PG
39 38 37 36
© Pan Books Ltd, 1976
ISBN 0 330 24651 8
Set, printed and bound in Great Britain by
Richard Clay Ltd, Bungay, Suffolk

Contents

Introduction
by Eileen Fowler

Sometimes I wonder whether we have the wrong approach to overweight, if we tend to take it for granted that those who suffer from this very contemporary problem are greedy, weak and stupid. I think there are often deep-seated reasons for compulsive eating, that it acts like a drug, and is some form of escapism. But whether the tendencies are inherited or acquired, indulging one's love of food can be extremely dangerous.

This we know, and when excessive weight makes life uncomfortable, we usually do something about it, but it's a great deal easier and safer to control if it's recognized in the early stages. For instance, you hear someone murmur confidentially, 'I'm beginning to get a spare tyre round my waist. It's not what I eat, you know. I cannot understand it: I'm not doing anything different.' But they are – we all are. Times have changed, and as we approach the forties and fifties we tend to take more interest in food and less in exercise.

Take a look around you at your family and friends, and you'll see what I mean. No longer the walk after the evening meal. There's something you want to see on television – anyway there's a car outside if you must go out. Our friends, bless them, ask us to dinner, remembering all our favourite dishes and little weaknesses. Misplaced kindness, but what can you say? Just smile and thank them and slide a little further forward on the bathroom scales.

But it isn't good enough, is it? We are jeopardizing our health, our looks and our energy. It's so insidious, this weight gathering: just a few extra calories a month and you are quite a bit heavier by Christmas.

However, our bodies have their own way of paying us back when we over-indulge at the festive season, making sure we know that we've offended. Headaches, indigestion and a bloated feeling leave us in no doubt that a little discretion would have made us feel better and left us a little slimmer. The trouble is the more you eat the more you can eat, and the less you eat the less interested you are in food. All this gets you nowhere. You must eat regularly and according to your needs, but for every good reason under the sun, it should be the right kind of food and the right quantity.

Goodness knows, it isn't always our fault if we have to battle with the bulge. Lots of figure problems are occupational. Think how often we have to stoop, sagging at shoulders and chest: washing-up, ironing, bathing the baby, working at desk or bench. We start with occupational hazards that leave us with slack muscles just asking for a coating of fat. The one-time sportsman, used to much muscular effort, often has time no longer for his regular exercise once he is married: his wife is a good cook – so here we go again.

So why don't we take a good look in that long mirror – all alone, mind, with nobody near enough to say, 'What are you worrying about? I like you that way – you're so cuddly.' Now that's all very well, but do you like yourself that way? It's what matters, because in five years' time, you won't be just cuddly, you'll be overweight. Figures don't stay the way you want them to; in most cases they tend to thicken and get set as the years go by and only sensible eating and exercise win the battle against time.

But it's not easy, especially for the men. Giving up smoking, business worries, less time to keep themselves fit make it difficult – just when a young and slim appearance is such an advantage.

What sort of shape is your husband in? You can't force a man to do a bit of good for himself, but you can persuade, drop hints, and quietly nudge him along the right road, and what better example than yourself? The way to a man's heart isn't through his stomach unless it's the right way, especially if he has to face up to business entertainment.

Another fallacy is this 'fat and happy' label. I've seen more than enough hidden tension in the overweight. *Relaxed* and *happy, yes* – at least you won't be over-eating or drinking too much to quieten your nerves. If you suffer this way, try walking. Yes, I know you've heard all this before, but have you really tried it? Not a short stroll round the park but walking in the exercise sense. Comfortable shoes, and your arms empty and free to swing make it a pleasure and not a chore.

Don't worry too much about the weather; as it becomes a habit you'll get stronger and better able to face up to a stiff breeze or a summer shower. Avoid north-east winds and a soaking downpour, but be properly equipped, just in case. Even if your surroundings as you walk are not exactly ideal, at least you are making your body work and this is what it needs. You don't age because of what you do in this way, but because of what you don't do. I have this on the highest scientific authority. Walking automatically deepens your breathing, cleanses the bloodstream and makes hundreds of muscles move, and the tension gradually lessens. This has been my personal experience and I can thoroughly recommend it.

So what's the answer to it all? I think the answer lies within ourselves. Do we want to keep reasonably slim, healthy and energetic, fit for what we have to do and want to do, or is the price too high to pay? It's as simple as that. You see, I believe that we can achieve anything within reason if we make up our minds that it's all worth while. It's literally a question of mind over matter. Why should we be permanently on the defensive against the gibes of our slimmer acquaintances when we can feel well, happy and confident by counting our calories and seeing that our leisure is active?

Perhaps you are thinking – yes, that's all very well, but how boring. Well, at first, maybe, but not if you've ever experienced or even seen the joy that emanates from those who stop slumping and regain their figure, good posture and one hundred per cent efficiency – to say nothing of the loss of double chins, huge upper arms, and legs and ankles that swell.

Group therapy has many advantages for those who wish to slim, just as attending a Keep Fit class makes the going faster. But not everyone has the time to spare or it may not be convenient. So count your calories at home, at work and play. Let's do it – all of us at the same time – as we read this book.

Best wishes,
Eileen Fowler

Note

The calorific values calculated for this book are taken
from 'The Composition of Foods', Medical Research
Council SRS 297, by R. A. McCance and
E. M. Widdowson, issued by
Her Majesty's Stationery Office.

The value of calorie counting

Calorie counting is probably the easiest and most popular method of weight control. A calorie is a unit of energy. The body uses up these units of energy, so when you take as many calorific units a day as you use up in energy, your weight should remain constant. However, if your intake is 2,500 and your expenditure is 2,000, you have a calorific excess of 500 units, which, in time, represents something like 50 grammes (2 oz) of solid fat. It is very difficult to estimate exactly how much energy we use up during a day. Obviously, someone doing manual labour all day long will use more than a person sitting at an office desk. An average thirty-year old man needs between 2,500 and 3,500 calorific units a day, whereas a woman will use up only between 1,750 and 2,250. As you grow older, you need fewer calories per day – from about the age of twenty-five.

One of the first things to remember when you go on a diet is that you will lose more weight in the first week than in the subsequent ones, because you should be losing extra liquid from your body as well as breaking down fat. To break down the fat cells in your body (which is how you really lose weight and your shape can change), you need to expend more energy per day than you absorb in calorific units through food. If you eat approximately 250 calories less than you use up, then you should break down 25 grammes (1 oz) of solid fat; if the difference is 500 calories, then 50 grammes (2 oz) of fat will be used up from your body's store of fat, and so on.

It is unwise to go on a crash diet of bananas and water or grapefruit and boiled eggs or any other diet advocating that you lose 3.5 kilogrammes (8 lb) during a week. Not only is it bad for your health generally, so that you become run down (and so more susceptible to minor ailments such as colds and coughs, etc) but you become very bored with eating the same consistency of food – which means that at the end of the diet, your yearning for a baked potato filled with butter, or half a pound of salted peanuts will be increased. On short diets, too, say for a week or two, most of the weight loss results from dehydration of the body system (losing extra water) so that in fact you have not lost any fat at all. So, when you return to your normal daily diet, absorbing the same amount of fluid, your weight will return to what it was immediately before the diet.

The best way to start reducing your weight is to set a limit on calorific intake for a couple of weeks – if you are a woman, say, 1,500 and if you are a man, say, 2,250. At the end of each week, you should have lost approximately 225 grammes (½ lb). If after two weeks, you find that you have not lost weight, then you obviously use up less energy than the 1,500 or 2,250 calorific units you are taking in – or you are forgetting the odd doughnut you bought by mistake... You should try reducing your intake of calories by a further 250 units per day. Or, if you want to lose weight at a faster rate than 225 grammes (½ lb), you could reduce your calorific intake to, say, 1,000 or 1,750, so that you should lose about 675–900 grammes (1½–2 lb) of solid fat per week. A calorific deficit of 1,000 units means that you'll lose 450 grammes (1 lb) in four days or about 3.5 kilogrammes (8 lb) in a month. You should not enlarge your calorific deficit beyond 1,000 units per day without consulting your doctor.

Each type of food – fat, protein, carbohydrate – converts to solid fat which is stored around the body. Each is essential to a healthy diet. It is unwise, therefore, to cut out all carbohydrates and fats just because they have higher calorie counts, leaving your intake to consist merely of protein such as meat, if you want a well-balanced and healthy diet. Cut down on fatty foods and carbohydrates, but don't exclude them altogether.

There are one or two points worth making about how you spread your calorific intake throughout the day. It is generally thought that one good big meal a day is sufficient, when taken in conjunction with breakfast, tea and a light lunch or dinner, depending on when you have your main meal. Sometimes you may be entertaining friends or going out for a meal and it may be difficult to limit your calorie intake. However, over the week, you can make adjustments so that, say, at weekends you are allowed two or three hundred more calories than on weekdays. But don't have 5,000 calories one day out of a weekly allowance of, say, 7,000 per week and starve yourself for the rest of the period.

Some people tend to want snacks throughout the day – well, it is thought that small meals, taken often, make weight loss easier, and as long as you keep a strict count of all your snacks and make sure they contain the right mixture of carbohydrate, fat and protein, you should be successful.

It is worth bearing in mind that if you have a large meal in the evening, you will be slightly more likely to put on extra pounds than if you have a large meal in the middle of the day; this is because, if you go to bed soon after a big meal, you will have less chance of using up the calories than if you have an afternoon and evening of activity to use up the energy. Even if you stay in bed all day, you still require about 1,000 calorific units.

You will not find it encouraging to rush into the bathroom each morning to find out how much weight you've lost the previous day. It is best to weigh yourself once a week – and if you do it in the morning after you have been to the lavatory, you will be at your lightest. Keep a weekly chart of your progress – this is one of the best encouragements to keep you from breaking the diet. Chart your present weight and the weight you want to reach and fill it in once a week.

This all boils down to one basic factor – *if you want to lose weight you must eat less,* which is the same as saying you must reduce your intake of calories. Keep counting calories, be sensible about it and you should be able to keep to your right weight.

What you should weigh

Obviously this is only an approximate guide and is simply
to give you some sort of target to work to. If you weigh
yourself with clothes, then deduct about 2 pounds
from your weight as shown on the chart which follows.
These weights are given for those over 25; deduct 1 pound
for each year under 25 if you are between 18 and 24.

Women

Height ft in	Small frame st lb	Medium frame st lb	Large frame st lb
4 10	6 11	7 3	7 13
4 11	6 13	7 6	8 2
5 0	7 2	7 9	8 5
5 1	7 5	7 12	8 8
5 2	7 8	8 1	8 11
5 3	7 11	8 4	9 0
5 4	8 0	8 7	9 3
5 5	8 4	8 11	9 7
5 6	8 6	9 1	9 11
5 7	8 10	9 5	10 1
5 8	9 0	9 9	10 5
5 9	9 4	9 13	10 9
5 10	9 9	10 3	11 0
5 11	9 13	10 7	11 4
6 0	10 5	10 11	11 9

Men

Height ft in	Small frame st lb	Medium frame st lb	Large frame st lb
5 2	8 4	8 11	9 7
5 3	8 7	9 1	9 10
5 4	8 10	9 4	10 0
5 5	8 13	9 7	10 3
5 6	9 2	9 10	10 7
5 7	9 6	10 0	10 11
5 8	9 10	10 5	11 2
5 9	10 0	10 9	11 6
5 10	10 5	10 13	11 10
5 11	10 9	11 3	12 1
6 0	10 13	11 8	12 6
6 1	11 3	11 12	12 10
6 2	11 7	12 3	13 1
6 3	11 11	12 8	13 6
6 4	12 1	12 13	13 11

Calorie counter

This chart gives the approximate calorific values
for 1 ounce and 100 grammes of the particular food.
(Both figures have been given to the nearest whole
number.)

	per oz	per 100g
All-Bran (Kelloggs)	80	311
Almonds, shelled	170	598
Anchovies	40	141
Apple dumpling	57	202
Apple pie	54	190
Apple pudding	68	239
Apples, eating, weighed with skin and core	10	36
Apples, cooking, baked	9	31
Apples, cooking, stewed without sugar	9	28
Apples, imported, eating	13	47
Apricots, fresh, weighed with stone	7	26
Apricots, fresh, stewed without sugar	6	22
Apricots, dried, raw	52	183
Apricots, dried, stewed without sugar	17	61
Apricots, tinned in syrup	30	106
Arrowroot	101	355
Artichokes, globe, boiled	2	7
Artichokes, Jerusalem, boiled	5	19
Asparagus, boiled	3	9
Asparagus, tinned or frozen	5	18
Avocado pear, weighed without stone	25	88

	per oz	per 100g
Bacon, raw	115	405
Bacon, fried	169	597
Bacon, gammon, fried	126	444
Bacon, streaky, fried	149	526
Bananas, weighed with skin	13	45
Banana custard	29	103
Barley, pearl, raw	102	360
Barley, pearl, boiled	34	120
Bass, steamed, weighed with bones	19	67
Beans, baked (Heinz)	26	93
Beans, broad, boiled	12	43
Beans, butter, boiled	26	93
Beans, French, boiled	2	7
Beans, haricot, boiled	25	89
Beans, runner, boiled	2	7
Beef, corned	66	231
Beef, roast sirloin, lean and fat	64	385
Beef, silverside, boiled	86	301
Beef, steak, raw	50	177
Beef, steak, fried	78	273
Beef, steak, grilled	86	304
Beef, steak, stewed	58	206
Beef, steak pudding	74	261
Beef, topside, boiled	61	213
Beef, topside, roast, lean and fat	91	321
Beef stew	40	140
Beefburger, frozen	70	246
Beetroot, boiled	13	44
Bemax	105	368
Biscuits, cream crackers	127	447
Biscuits, digestive	137	481

	per oz	per 100g
Biscuits, plain, mixed	123	435
Biscuits, rusks	116	409
Biscuits, sweet	158	556
Biscuits, water	126	444
Blackberries, raw	8	30
Blackberries, stewed without sugar	6	23
Blancmange	34	118
Bloaters, grilled, weighed with bones and skin	54	189
Boiled sweets	93	327
Bounty Bars	137	481
Bournvita	105	370
Bovril	23	80
Brain, calf, boiled	29	103
Brain, sheep, boiled	31	110
Branston pickle	37	130
Brazil nuts, weighed with shells	82	289
Bread, Allinsons	65	228
Bread, brown	68	242
Bread, currant	71	252
Bread, Hovis	67	237
Bread, malt	71	250
Bread, Procea	72	255
Bread, large white	69	243
Bread, white, fried	162	569
Bread, white, toasted	85	299
Bread, wholemeal	65	229
Breadcrumbs, dried	101	355
Bread sauce	32	112
Bread-and-butter pudding	46	162
Bream, red, steamed with bones	17	61

	per oz	per 100g
Bream, sea, steamed with bones	19	66
Brill, steamed with bones	22	78
Broccoli, boiled	4	14
Brown sauce, bottled	28	115
Brussels sprouts, raw	9	32
Brussels sprouts, boiled	5	16
Butter, slightly salted	226	793
Buck rarebit	81	287

	per oz	per 100g
Cabbage, red, raw	6	20
Cabbage, Savoy, boiled	3	9
Cabbage, Spring, boiled	2	8
Canary pudding	131	461
Carrots, raw	6	23
Carrots, young, boiled	6	21
Carrots, tinned, Smedleys	5	19
Cashew nuts	178	626
Castle pudding	112	394
Catfish, steamed, with bones	28	100
Catfish, fried in batter	53	188
Cauliflower, raw	7	25
Cauliflower, boiled	3	11
Celeriac, boiled	4	14
Celery, raw	3	9
Celery, boiled	1	5
Cheese, Camembert	88	313
Cheese, Cheddar	120	424
Cheese, cottage	33	116
Cheese, cream	230	809
Cheese, Danish Blue	103	366
Cheese, Edam	88	313
Cheese, Gorgonzola	112	393
Cheese, Gouda	96	340
Cheese, Jarlsberg	95	334
Cheese, Mysot	133	468
Cheese, Parmesan	118	420
Cheese, processed	106	374
Cheese, spread	82	290
Cheese, St Ivel	108	380
Cheese, Stilton	135	477

	per oz	per 100g
Cheese, Wensleydale	115	406
Cheese straws	102	359
Chef sauce	28	99
Cherry cake	129	454
Cherries, eating, weighed with stones	11	40
Cherries, stewed, without sugar	10	35
Cherries, glacé	60	212
Chestnuts, weighed in shells	40	141
Chicken, boiled, weighed with bones	38	132
Chicken, roast, weighed with bones	29	102
Chicken Noodle Soup Mix, Batchelors	95	334
Chicory, raw	3	9
Chocolate, milk	167	588
Chocolate, plain	155	544
Chocolate cake	141	496
Chocolate mould	35	123
Chutney, apple	57	201
Chutney, tomato	43	151
Cobnuts, weighed in shells	41	145
Cockles	13	48
Cocoa	128	452
Coconut, fresh	104	366
Coconut, desiccated	178	627
Cod, steamed, weighed with skin and bones	19	66
Cod, fried in batter, from shop	58	204
Cod, steak, grilled with butter	39	136
Cod's roe, fried	59	206
Cod's roe, baked in vinegar	34	128
Cod liver oil	264	930
Coffee, black	0	0

	per oz	per 100g
Consommé	4	14
Corn on the cob, tinned	20	70
Cornflakes, Kelloggs	104	367
Cornflour	100	354
Crab, boiled, weighed with shell	7	25
Cranberries, raw	4	15
Cucumber, raw	3	9
Currant bun	87	306
Currant cake	119	418
Currants, black, raw	8	29
Currants, black, stewed without sugar	6	22
Currants, red, raw	6	21
Currants, red, stewed without sugar	4	16
Currants, white, raw	7	26
Currants, white, stewed without sugar	6	20
Curry, without rice	48	169
Curry powder	67	236
Custard powder	see cornflour	
Custard powder, boiled	33	116
Custard tart	82	289

	per oz	per 100g
Dabs, fried, weighed with bones	56	199
Damsons, raw, weighed with stones	9	34
Damsons, stewed without sugar	8	29
Dates, weighed with stones	61	214
Dogfish, fried, weighed with bones	85	300
Doughnuts	101	355
Dripping, beef	262	920
Duck, roast, weighed with bones	48	169
Dumpling	59	206
Dundee Cake	110	389

	per oz	per 100g
Easter biscuits	134	473
Eccles cakes	147	518
Eel, Conger, fried, weighed with bones	72	252
Eel, Conger, steamed, weighed with bones	23	83
Eel, silver, stewed	106	374
Eggplant (aubergine), raw	4	15
Egg custard, baked	32	113
Egg custard, sauce	34	119
Egg sauce	42	148
Eggs, whole	46	163
Eggs, whites	11	39
Eggs, yolks	99	350
Eggs, boiled	55	193
Eggs, fried	68	240
Eggs, poached	45	159
Eggs, scotch	75	265
Eggs, scrambled	79	279
Endive, raw	3	11
Energen	111	390

	per oz	per 100 g
Familia Muesli	104	366
Farex	97	348
Fig rolls	110	387
Figs, green	12	41
Figs, dried, raw	61	214
Fishcakes	61	215
Fish Fingers	50	176
Fish paste	49	174
Flounder, steamed, weighed with skin and bones	15	53
Flounder, fried, weighed with skin and bones	42	147
Flour, English, 100%	95	333
Flour, English, 80%	99	348
Flour, English, Patent	100	352
Flour, Manitoba, 100%	96	339
Flour, Manitoba, 80%	99	350
Flour, Manitoba, Patent	100	351
Flour, rye, 100%	95	335
Flour, rye, 60%	101	350
Flour, wholemeal	95	334
Fruit gums, Rowntree's	49	171
Fruit Salad, canned in syrup	27	94
Fudge	120	422

	per oz	per 100g
Ginger, ground	74	259
Ginger biscuits	127	447
Gingerbread	108	381
Glucose, Liquid BP	90	318
Goose, roast, weighed with bones	53	187
Grapenuts	102	358
Grapes, whole, raw, black	14	51
Grapes, whole, raw, white	17	60
Grapefruit, raw	3	11
Grapefruit squash	39	136
Greengages, weighed with stones	13	45
Greengages, weighed with stones, stewed without sugar	11	37
Grouse, roast, weighed with bones	32	114
Guinea-fowl, roast, weighed with bones	32	114

	per oz	per 100g
Haddock, fried, weighed with skin and bones	55	193
Haddock, smoked, steamed, weighed with skin and bones	28	65
Hake, fried, weighed with skin and bones	55	193
Hake, steamed, weighed with skin and bones	24	86
Halibut, steamed weighed with skin and bones	28	99
Ham, York, boiled, lean only	62	219
Ham, York, boiled, lean and fat	123	435
Hare, roast	55	193
Hare, stewed or baked	55	194
Heart, sheep, roast	68	239
Herring, fried, weighed with skin and bones	59	208
Herring, baked in vinegar, weighed with skin and bones	50	174
Herring roe, fried	74	260
Honey	82	288
Honeycomb	80	281
Horlicks Malted Milk	113	399
Horseradish, raw	17	60

	per oz	per 100g
Ice cream, chocolate	80	282
Ice cream, coffee	68	239
Ice cream, vanilla	56	196
Imperial biscuits	133	468
Irish Stew	42	147
Jams, stoned fruit	74	261
Jam tarts	112	394
Jam roll, baked	115	403
Jelly	23	82
Jelly, milk	31	111
John Dory, steamed, weighed with skin and bones	17	59
Kedgeree	43	152
Kidney, ox, stewed	45	159
Kidney, sheep, fried	57	199
Kippers, grilled or baked, weighed with skin and bones	31	108

	per oz	per 100g
Lamb chop, grilled, weighed with bone	108	378
Lamb chop, fried, weighed with bone	146	512
Lamb, leg of, roast	74	292
Lamb, neck of, stewed, weighed with bone	69	245
Lard	262	920
Leeks, raw	9	30
Leeks, boiled	7	25
Leicester pudding	102	358
Lemon	4	15
Lemon curd	86	302
Lemon curd tarts	125	442
Lemon juice	2	7
Lemon squash	36	126
Lemonade	6	21
Lentils, boiled	27	96
Lentil soup	29	100
Lettuce, raw	3	11
Lime juice cordial	32	112
Ling, fried, weighed with skin and bones	52	185
Liquorice Allsorts	90	315
Liver, calf, fried	74	262
Liver, ox, fried	71	254
Liver sausage	97	341
Lobster, boiled, weighed in shell	12	43
Loganberries, raw	5	17
Loganberries, stewed without sugar	4	13
Loganberries, tinned	29	101
Lucozade	19	67
Luncheon meat, tinned	95	335

	per oz	per 100g
Macaroni, boiled	32	114
Macaroni cheese	59	207
Mackerel, fried, weighed with skin and bones	39	136
Mandarins, tinned	18	64
Margarine	226	795
Marmalade	74	216
Marmite	2	6
Marrow, boiled	2	7
Mars Bars	127	447
Meat paste	61	215
Medlars, weighed with skin and stones	10	34
Melon, Cantaloupe, whole	4	15
Melon, Yellow, whole	4	13
Milk, fresh	19	66
Milk, fresh, skimmed	10	35
Milk, condensed, sweetened	100	354
Milk, condensed, unsweetened	45	159
Milk, dried	150	530
Milk, dried, skimmed	93	326
Mincemeat	37	129
Mince pies	111	393
Minestrone	18	63
Mixed fruit pudding	92	325
Monkfish, steamed, weighed with skin and bones	23	79
Monkfish, fried, weighed with skin and bones	41	145
Mulberries, raw	10	36
Mullet, red and grey, steamed, weighed with skin and bones	23	85

	per oz	per 100g
Mushrooms, raw	2	7
Mushrooms, fried	62	217
Mussels, boiled	25	87
Mussels, boiled, weighed in shells	7	26
Mustard powder	132	463
Mustard-and-cress, raw	3	10
Nectarines, weighed with stones	13	46
Nescafé, black	0	0
Nougat	122	429
Oatmeal, raw	115	404
Oatmeal porridge	13	45
Olives, in brine, weighed with stones	24	85
Olive oil	264	930
Omelette, plain	57	200
Omelette, jam	78	276
Onions, raw	7	23
Onions, boiled	4	13
Onions, fried	101	355
Onions, Spring, raw	10	36
Onion sauce	25	88
Orange, weighed with peel and pips	8	27
Orange cake, plain	132	465
Orange juice	11	38
Orange squash	39	136
Ostermilk, No 1	129	453
Ovaltine	109	384
Oxo cubes	33	116
Oysters, raw, in shells	2	6

	per oz	per 100g
Pancakes	85	301
Parsley	6	21
Parsnips, boiled	16	56
Partridge, roast, weighed with bones	36	127
Passionfruit, weighed with skin	4	15
Pastilles	73	254
Pastry, flaky, baked	167	589
Pastry, shortcrust, baked	157	548
Pâté	132	465
Peaches, weighed with stone	9	32
Peaches, dried, raw	61	213
Peaches, dried, stewed without sugar	20	70
Peaches, tinned in syrup	25	87
Peanuts	171	603
Peanut butter	180	634
Pears, imported eating, weighed with skin and core	8	29
Pears, English eating, weighed with skin and core	9	30
Pears, stewed without sugar	8	27
Pears, tinned in syrup	22	77
Peas, fresh, raw	18	64
Peas, fresh, boiled	14	49
Peas, dried, boiled	28	100
Peas, split, dried, boiled	33	116
Peas, tinned	24	86
Pemmican (Bovril)	167	590
Pepper	88	309
Peppermints, boiled	111	391
Pheasant, roast, weighed with bones	38	134
Piccalilli	7	25

	per oz	per 100g
Pigeon, boiled, weighed with bones	27	96
Pigeon, roast, weighed with bones	29	102
Pilchards, tinned, drained of oil	54	191
Pistachio nuts	168	591
Plaice, steamed, weighed with skin and bones	18	50
Plaice, fried in batter, weighed with skin and bones	40	145
Plain fruit cake	107	378
Plums, Victoria, weighed with stones	10	36
Plums, stewed without sugar, weighed with stones	6	20
Plum pie	52	183
Pollack, steamed, weighed with skin and bones	21	75
Pollack, steaks, fried in batter	41	145
Pollan, steamed, weighed with skin and bones	16	58
Pollan, fried in oatmeal	40	142
Pomegranate juice	13	44
Popcorn	137	482
Pork, leg of, roast	90	317
Pork, loin of, roast, lean only	81	284
Pork, loin of, roast, lean and fat	129	455
Pork chop, grilled, lean only, weighed with bone	38	133
Pork chop, grilled, lean and fat, weighed with bone	128	451
Pork pie	104	366
Potatoes, old, boiled	23	80
Potatoes, old, mashed with milk and margarine	34	120

	per oz	per 100g
Potatoes, old, jacket, weighed with skins	24	84
Potatoes, old, roast	35	123
Potatoes, old, chips	68	239
Potatoes, new, boiled	21	75
Potato soup	26	92
Potato Crisps, Smith's	159	559
Prawns	30	104
Prawns, weighed in shells	11	40
Prunes, dried, raw, weighed with stones	38	134
Prunes, stewed, without sugar, weighed with stones	19	81
Puffed Wheat	102	358
Pumpkin, raw	4	15
Queen of Puddings	60	213
Queen's Cake	129	455
Quinces	7	25
Rabbit, stewed, weighed with bones	26	92
Radishes	4	14
Raisins, dried	70	247
Raspberries, raw	7	25
Raspberries, stewed without sugar	7	23
Rhubarb, stewed without sugar	1	5
Rhubarb pie	53	229
Ribena	65	188
Rice, boiled	35	122
Rice pudding	42	144
Rice Krispies, Kelloggs	100	351
Rock cakes	119	418
Ryvita	98	345

	per oz	per 100g
Sago	101	355
Sago pudding	36	127
Saithe, steamed, weighed with skin and bones	24	83
Salad cream (Heinz)	111	387
Salmon, fresh, steamed, weighed with skin and bones	57	161
Salmon, tinned	39	137
Salsify, boiled	5	18
Salt, block and free-running	0	0
Sardines, tinned	84	294
Sausage, beef, fried	81	287
Sausage, pork, fried	93	326
Sausage, black	81	286
Sausage roll, flaky pastry	142	498
Sausage roll, shortcrust pastry	134	474
Scallops, steamed, weighed without shells	30	105
Scampi	85	299
Scones	105	369
Seakale, boiled	2	8
Semolina pudding	37	131
Shepherd's pie	32	114
Shortbread	148	521
Shredded Wheat	103	362
Shrimps	32	114
Skate, fried, weighed with bones	57	201
Smelts, fried, weighed whole	98	346
Sole, steamed, weighed with skin and bones	14	50
Sole, fried, weighed with skin and bones	68	241

	per oz	per 100g
Sole, Lemon, steamed, weighed with skin and bones	18	64
Sole, Lemon, fried, weighed with skin and bones	49	173
Soya, low-fat flour	95	335
Spaghetti	104	365
Spaghetti, tinned in tomato sauce (Heinz)	17	60
Spinach, boiled	7	26
Sponge cake	87	308
Sprats, fresh, fried, weighed whole	111	390
Sprats, smoked, grilled, weighed whole	81	284
Spring greens, boiled	3	10
Stockfish, boiled, weighed with skin and bones	33	116
Strawberries, fresh	7	26
Sturgeon, steamed, weighed with bones	30	105
Suet	262	925
Suet pudding	105	370
Sugar, Demerara	112	394
Sugar, white	112	394
Sultanas	70	249
Swedes, boiled	5	18
Sweetbreads, stewed	51	178
Sweet potatoes, boiled	23	80
Swiss apple pudding	63	222
Syrup, golden	84	297
Syrup, sponge pudding	104	368

	per oz	per 100g
Tangerines, weighed with peel and pips	7	24
Tapioca	102	359
Tapioca pudding	37	129
Tartare sauce	80	282
Tea, Indian, without milk	0	0
Thick Pea Soup (Batchelors)	106	369
Toad-in-the-Hole	82	290
Toffees, mixed	123	435
Tomatoes, raw	4	14
Tomatoes, fried	20	71
Tomato juice	7	25
Tomato Ketchup	28	99
Tomato sauce	21	74
Tomato Soup (Heinz)	19	69
Tongue, ox, pickled	88	309
Tongue, sheep, stewed	84	297
Torsk, steamed, weighed with skin and bones	16	58
Torsk, fried, weighed with skin and bones	30	105
Treacle, black	73	257
Treacle tart	107	375
Trifle	43	150
Tripe, stewed	29	102
Trout, steamed, weighed with skin and bones	25	88
Trout, sea, steamed, weighed with skin and bones	29	104
Turbot, steamed, weighed with skin and bones	19	66

	per oz	per 100 g
Turkey, roast, weighed with bones	34	118
Turnips, boiled	3	11
Veal, cutlet, fried	61	216
Veal, fillet, roast	66	232
Vegetable soup, tinned (Heinz)	12	43
Venison, roast	56	197
Victoria sandwich cake	134	473
Vinegar	1	4
Virol	99	349
Vita-Weat	120	423

	per oz	per 100g
Walnuts, shelled	156	549
Walnuts, with shells	100	352
Watercress, raw	4	15
Water ice	20	70
Weetabix	100	351
Welsh cheese cakes	139	489
Welsh rarebit	102	358
Whelks, weighed with shells	4	14
White sauce, savoury	41	143
White sauce, sweet	47	165
Whitebait, fried, weighed whole	152	537
Whiting, steamed, weighed with skin and bones	17	61
Whiting, fried, weighed with skin and bones	49	174
Winkles, boiled in salt or fresh water, weighed with shells	4	14
Witch, steamed, weighed with skin and bones	15	53
Witch, fried, weighed with skin and bones	56	196
Yoghurt, low fat	15	54
Yoghurt, fruit	30	106
Yorkshire pudding	63	218

Alcohol and soft drinks

Beer	approx per pint	per fl oz	per 100 ml
Brown ale, bottled	160	8	28
Draught ale, bitter	180	9	31
Draught ale, mild	140	7	25
Pale ale, bottled	180	9	32
Stout, bottled	200	10	37
Stout, extra	220	11	39
Strong ale	420	21	73

Cider			
Dry	200	10	37
Sweet	240	12	42
Vintage	560	28	100

Wines	approx per glass		
Port, ruby	129	43	152
Port, tawny	135	45	160
Sherry, dry	99	33	114
Sherry, sweet	114	38	135
Champagne	105	21	74
Graves	105	21	73
Sauternes	130	26	93
Burgundy	100	20	72
Beaujolais	95	19	68
Chianti	90	18	65
Médoc	90	18	63

Spirits	per pub measure $\frac{1}{6}$th gill
Scotch whisky	58
Irish whiskey	63
Gin	55
Rum	75
Vodka	63

Soft drinks	12 oz tin	per fl oz	per 100 ml
Coca-Cola		12	41
Tab	·75	—	—
Lucozade		21	75
Bitter lemon		9	32
Dry ginger ale		4	14
Ginger beer		11	39
American ginger ale		11	39
Soda-water		—	—
Tonic water		6	21

Liqueurs	approx per glass
Benedictine	75
Brandy	75
Chartreuse	75
Cherry brandy	90
Crème de menthe	90
Curaçao	70
Drambuie	65
Kümmel	70

Low-calorie recipes

Starters

Soups can be divided into two groups: thin soups made with home-made stock and which contain no thickening ingredients such as cornflour or potato; and those which contain cream, egg yolks, flour or potatoes. Soups in the second category usually contain a large number of calories per portion and should be avoided by the calorie conscious; I will give some recipes for the first group.

Tomato soup

serves 4   calories per portion: 40

450 g (1 lb) tomatoes
1 large onion, finely sliced
1 clove garlic, crushed

1 tablespoon olive oil
6 dl (1 pint) chicken stock
salt and pepper to taste

Heat the oil in a large saucepan. Add the onion and garlic and fry until softened. Put the tomatoes in boiling water for thirty seconds, then remove the skins. Chop roughly and add to saucepan. Cook for 5 minutes over a low heat and then add the stock. Simmer for 15–20 minutes until the tomatoes are soft, then blend in an electric blender or put through a Mouli. Season with salt and pepper and serve piping hot, garnished with parsley or thin slices of lemon. This soup can also be served cold, in which case it should be chilled in the refrigerator for several hours.

Watercress soup

serves 4   calories per portion: 39

1 onion, finely sliced
2 bunches watercress
6 dl (1 pint) stock
3 dl (½ pint) milk made with 25 g (1 oz) dried low-fat milk
and 3 dl (½ pint) water
salt and pepper to taste
pinch nutmeg

Wash watercress and remove any tough stalks. Chop
roughly and reserve about half a bunch for decoration at
the end. Put watercress, onion and stock into a large
saucepan and bring to the boil. Simmer gently for 15–20
minutes, until the vegetables are tender. Stir in the milk,
and put through a Mouli or blend in an electric blender.
Adjust seasoning, add nutmeg and serve garnished with
remaining watercress. Serve hot or put in the refrigerator
to chill for several hours.

Consommé with yoghurt and lumpfish roe

serves 3   calories per portion: 55

1 tin Crosse & Blackwell's Consommé
1 small carton natural yoghurt
1 small pot Danish lumpfish roe
salt and pepper to taste

In a saucepan, gently heat the consommé until melted.
Season with salt and pepper and pour into individual
bowls. Put in refrigerator to set – this should take one to
two hours. Cover each portion with the yoghurt and then
sprinkle about 1 teaspoon of lumpfish roe evenly over
the yoghurt.

Melon balls with orange
serves 4   calories per portion: 65

1 ripe Honeydew melon
juice and grated rind of 1 orange
juice of ½ lemon

Cut the melon in half and remove the seeds. Using a round
vegetable scoop, cut the melon into round balls. Put them
into a large bowl, and mix in the fruit juices and grated
orange rind. Allow to chill for several hours and serve in
individual bowls.

Moules Marinière
serves 4   calories per portion: 60

Mussels are very cheap when in season (roughly from
September until April), and although they take a
considerable time to clean they do have a reasonably low
calorific value.

1 gallon mussels
1 tablespoon olive oil
1 onion, finely sliced
1 clove garlic, crushed
6 dl (1 pint) stock

Clean the mussels and remove the beards. Discard any
which are open or which feel very heavy – they may
contain mud. Rinse them two or three times in cold water.
In a large saucepan, heat the oil and add the onion and
garlic. Fry gently until softened and pour in the stock.
Bring to the boil and add the mussels. Shake the pan and
leave to boil vigorously for 2–3 minutes, by which time
the mussels should have opened. Serve in soup bowls with
the liquid. Any mussels which have not opened during the
cooking stage should be discarded.

Salads and main courses

Salade Niçoise

serves 4   calories per portion: 85

2 hard-boiled eggs
2 ripe tomatoes
8 good lettuce leaves
8–10 anchovy fillets

8–10 black olives, stoned
50 g (2 oz) tuna fish
4 tablespoons vinegar
or lemon juice

Shell the eggs and cut them into quarters. Put the
tomatoes in boiling water for 30 seconds and remove the
skins. Slice thinly. Arrange the lettuce leaves on four
plates, then the eggs and tomatoes. Flake the well-drained
tuna fish, arrange on the salads, decorate with the anchovy
fillets and olives and pour over the vinegar or lemon juice.

Cottage cheese and cucumber salad

serves 4   calories per portion: 75

225 g (8 oz) cottage cheese
1 cucumber, finely diced
8–10 black olives, stoned
8 good lettuce leaves
4 tablespoons vinegar or lemon juice
salt and pepper to taste
2 tablespoons chives

In a bowl, mix the cottage cheese with the cucumber and
chives. Season with salt and pepper. Arrange the lettuce
leaves on four plates, and put a quarter of the mixture on
each plate. Decorate with the olives and pour over the
dressing of vinegar or lemon juice.

Broad bean and anchovy salad

serves 4   calories per portion: 101

225 g (8 oz) young broad beans
8–10 anchovy fillets
3 hard-boiled eggs
2 tablespoons chives, finely chopped
1·5 dl (¼ pint) tomato juice
1 tablespoon lemon juice
salt and pepper to taste
8 good lettuce leaves

Cook the broad beans in boiling salted water until tender.
Drain and leave to cool. Shell the eggs and cut into quarters.
Arrange lettuce leaves, broad beans and eggs on four
separate plates. Mix the tomato juice, lemon juice and salt
and pepper well and pour over the salads. Sprinkle with
chives.

Eggs with spinach

serves 4   calories per portion: 115

450 g (1 lb) spinach
4 eggs
salt and pepper to taste

Wash the spinach and discard any tough leaves. Boil it in a
large saucepan with 1·5 dl (¼ pint) water for 15 minutes or
until tender, and drain well. Put the spinach into a large
ovenproof dish, shape four holes in it and break an egg into
each hole. Put it into a pre-heated oven (175°C, 350°F,
Gas 4) for about 10 minutes or until the eggs are just set.
Season with salt and pepper and serve.

Savoury tomatoes

serves 4   calories per portion: 110

4 large tomatoes
50 g (2 oz) cold meat (ham or chicken)
1 small onion, finely sliced
50 g (2 oz) grated Cheddar cheese
salt and pepper to taste

Cut the tops off the tomatoes, scoop out the insides and mix them in a bowl with the finely chopped cold meat and the onion. Add the cheese and season. Spoon the mixture back into the tomatoes, replace the tops and bake in a moderate oven (175°C, 350°F, Gas 4) for 30 minutes.

Kedgeree

serves 3   calories per portion: 287

225 g (8 oz) smoked haddock, steamed
50 g (2 oz) rice
25 g (1 oz) margarine
1 hard-boiled egg
1 egg
salt and pepper to taste

Boil the rice in 1½ cupfuls of salted water for 15 minutes or until cooked. Drain and add to another saucepan in which you have melted the margarine. Add the flaked fish, the egg, beaten, and season with salt and pepper. Mix well and add the chopped hard-boiled egg. Turn the mixture into a well-greased pie dish and bake in a moderate oven (175°C, 350°F, Gas 4) for 20 minutes.

Grilled steak with lemon

serves 2   calories per portion: 328

2 steaks, approximately 170 g (6 oz) each
25 g (1 oz) margarine
freshly ground black pepper
½ lemon

Trim any excess fat off the steaks and season them with
pepper. Heat the grill until really hot. Lay the steaks on the
grill rack, dot with margarine and grill for 3–8 minutes on
each side depending on how rare you like them. Serve with
quarters of lemon.

Grilled trout with lemon

serves 2   calories per portion: 154

2 trout, approximately 340 g (12 oz) each
salt and freshly ground black pepper
1 tablespoon parsley, finely chopped
½ lemon

Clean the fish, slit open and remove the innards. Whether
you leave the head on or not is up to you; some people are
put off by it and others think it makes the fish look better.
Cut two or three gashes in the sides of the fish to allow the
heat to get through to the bone. Season both inside and
outside of the fish and put under a hot grill for about 6–7
minutes on each side. Decorate the wounds of the fish with
parsley and serve piping hot with quarters of lemon.

Beef casserole

serves 4   calories per portion: 424

25 g (1 oz) butter
1 onion, finely sliced
1 clove garlic, crushed
450 g (1 lb) stewing steak
6 dl (1 pint) good stock
50 g (2 oz) mushrooms
450 g (1 lb) carrots
salt and pepper

Melt half the butter in a large pan, add the onion and garlic
and cook until soft. Add the meat, cut up into small cubes
and continue to cook until the meat is browned on all
sides. Peel the carrots, slice lengthwise and add to the pan,
together with the stock. Cook in a moderate oven (160°C,
325°F, Gas 3) for about 1½ hours. Remove pan and add
sliced mushrooms that have previously been cooked in the
remaining butter. Return pan to oven and continue to
cook for half an hour or until the meat is fork-tender.
Adjust seasoning and serve.

Vegetable pie

serves 3   calories per portion: 204

100 g (4 oz) mushrooms
2 large onions, finely sliced
white of 1 leek, finely shredded
2 large aubergines, cut into slices
225 g (8 oz) tomatoes
salt and pepper to taste
25 g (1 oz) butter
2 tablespoons water

Sprinkle the aubergine slices with salt and allow to sweat
for half an hour. Drain well on kitchen paper. Stand the
tomatoes in boiling water for thirty seconds, then remove
the skins. Slice them and the mushrooms. Lightly grease a
casserole, line it with aubergine slices, followed by layers
of mushroom, tomato, leek and onion. Repeat until all
the ingredients are used up, finishing with a layer of
aubergine. Sprinkle with the cheese, dot with butter and
add the water. Bake in a moderate oven (175°C, 350°F,
Gas 4) for 1–1½ hours.

Chicken casserole

serves 4   calories per portion: 365

50 g (2 oz) butter
1 large onion, finely sliced
1 clove garlic, crushed
1 chicken, approximately 1 kg (2¼ lb)
1 tablespoonful chopped tarragon
100 g (4 oz) mushrooms
6 dl (1 pint) chicken stock
1 small glass white wine
salt and pepper to taste

Melt half the butter in a frying pan, add the onions and garlic and fry until softened but not brown. Transfer to casserole dish. Add remaining butter to frying pan and add chicken, cut up into joints. Brown on all sides, and put into casserole dish. Pour over stock, white wine, tarragon and season with salt and pepper. Put into a moderate oven (175°C, 350°F, Gas 4) for 1 hour. Remove and add mushrooms. Continue to cook for a further 30 minutes or until the meat is fork-tender.

Cabbage leaves stuffed with minced meat

serves 4   calories per portion: 209

450 g (1 lb) minced meat
1 large onion, finely chopped
1 clove garlic, crushed
1 tablespoon chopped parsley
8 large or 12 small cabbage leaves
3 dl (½ pint) chicken stock
salt and pepper to taste

Wash the cabbage leaves and boil them in lightly salted water for about five minutes. While you are doing this, mix the meat, onion, garlic and parsley in a large bowl and season well. Drain the cabbage leaves and fill them with the meat mixture. Roll them up and secure each with a cocktail stick. Place in a lightly greased baking dish and pour over the stock. Bake in a moderate oven (175°C, 350°F, Gas 4) for forty-five minutes.

Puddings

Raspberry mousse

serves 4   calories per portion: 110

450 g (1 lb) raspberries
liquid sweetener to taste
2 tablespoons water
4 egg whites

In a large saucepan, boil the raspberries with the sweetener
and water until pulpy – about five minutes. Put them
through a Mouli or blend in an electric blender, to make a
puree. Whisk the egg whites stiff and fold them into the
fruit. Reserve a few raspberries to decorate. Chill for
several hours.

Spiced oranges

serves 4   calories per portion: 50

4 large oranges
4.5 dl (¾ pint) water
½ teaspoon ground cinnamon
¼ teaspoon freshly ground nutmeg
liquid sweetener

Peel the oranges and remove all the white pith. Cut them
into slices. In a saucepan, heat the water and spices until
boiling point and add the orange slices. Simmer very
gently for three to four minutes. Add liquid sweetener if
desired. Leave to cool, then chill in the refrigerator for
several hours.

Pears in red wine

serves 4   calories per portion: 90

4 large ripe pears
½ teaspoon ground cinnamon
½ teaspoon freshly ground nutmeg
liquid sweetener
4.5 dl (¾ pint) red cooking wine

Peel the pears, leaving the stalks on and the pears whole. In a large saucepan, heat the spices, 3–4 drops of liquid sweetener and the red wine to boiling point. Add the pears and leave to simmer very gently for 30–45 minutes until the pears are tender. Either serve hot or allow to cool and chill in the refrigerator for several hours.

Rhubarb crumble

serves 4   calories per portion: 190

675 g (1½ lb) rhubarb	25 g (1 oz) butter
3–4 tablespoons water	50 g (2 oz) sugar
liquid sweetener	75 g (3 oz) flour

Cut the rhubarb into 2.5 cm (1″) slices and put into a saucepan with the water and 3–4 drops of sweetener. You may need more depending on how sweet you like your rhubarb. Bring to the boil and then turn heat as low as possible, or cook in the oven (140°C, 275°F, Gas 1), covered with a lid, for about fifteen minutes. Pour into a lightly greased ovenproof dish. Make the crumble by mixing the butter, sugar and flour until the butter is all broken down. Put the mixture on top of the rhubarb (if the rhubarb seems very liquid, remove some of the juice). Bake in a moderate oven (175°C, 350°F, Gas 4) for 15–20 minutes by which time the top should be lightly browned. There should be just enough crumble for everyone to have a taste.

Apple meringue

serves 4   calories per portion: 107

675 g (1½ lb) cooking apples
3–4 tablespoons water
liquid sweetener
4 egg whites

Peel and core the apples. Cut them into slices and place in a
saucepan with the water and liquid sweetener. Bring to the
boil and simmer very gently for 20–30 minutes, then pour
into a lightly greased ovenproof dish. Add a few drops of
sweetener to the egg whites and beat them until stiff.
Cover the apple with the beaten egg whites and bake in a
cool oven (150°C, 300°F, Gas 2) for about twenty minutes.

Blackberry fool

serves 4   calories per portion: 70

450 g (1 lb) ripe blackberries
3–4 tablespoons water
liquid sweetener
2 small cartons natural yoghurt

Wash the blackberries well and cook in a large saucepan
with the water and a few drops of liquid sweetener for
about 8–10 minutes or until tender. Put through an electric
blender or Mouli to form a pulp. Test for sweetness and
add more sweetener if necessary. Allow to cool and stir in
the yoghurt. Serve chilled.

Easy calculation of calories

For easy calculation of calorific content,
the average helping of the following is
equal to approximately the calories given:

All-Bran (Kelloggs)	100
Apricots, tinned	150
Avocado (½)	100
Bacon, two rashers, fried	350
Baked Beans	200
Beef, corned	250
Beef, roast	250
Beef, steak-and-kidney pudding	500
Beef, steak, grilled	325
Blancmange	150
Bournvita	50
Bream, red	100
Cheese, Camembert	100
Cheese, Cheddar	125
Cheese, Stilton	150
Cod, fried	250
Cornflakes	100
Custard, made with powder	100
Doughnuts	200
Duck, roast	350
Eggs, Scotch (1)	300
Eggs, scrambled (2)	200
Fruit jelly	100

Fruit salad	100
Gooseberry pie	300
Haddock, fried	300
Ham, boiled	400
Jam roll, baked	450
Kedgeree	150
Kipper (1)	200
Liver, fried	300
Luncheon meat	400
Mackerel, fried	300
Mince pies	150
Mussels	100
Orange (1)	50
Peach, fresh	50
Peas, fresh, boiled	50
Plaice, fried	400
Pork chop, grilled	600
Porridge	100
Potatoes, baked	100
Potatoes, chipped, fried	300
Potatoes, new, boiled	100
Rice Krispies	100
Sausages, pork, fried	200
Shepherd's pie	250
Shredded Wheat	100
Sole, fried	400
Spinach, boiled	25
Sponge pudding with syrup	400
Suet pudding	400
Toad-in-the-Hole	500
Treacle tart	400
Turkey, roast	225
Vita-Weat	100
Welsh rarebit	300
Yoghurt, fruit	150